WATER
INFUSIONS

WATER INFUSIONS

Refreshing, Detoxifying and Healthy Recipes for Your HOME INFUSER

MARIZA SNYDER & LAUREN CLUM

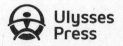

Ulysses Press

Published in the U.S. by
ULYSSES PRESS
P.O. Box 3440
Berkeley, CA 94703
www.ulyssespress.com

ISBN: 978-1-61243-401-8
Library of Congress Control Number 2014943041

Acquisitions Editor: Kelly Reed
Managing Editor: Claire Chun
Editor: Renee Rutledge
Proofreader: Lauren Harrison
Front cover/interior design and layout: what!design @ whatweb.com
Cover photo: © dashkin14/shutterstock.com

Printed in Canada by Marquis Book Printing

10 9 8 7 6 5 4 3 2 1

Distributed by Publishers Group West

NOTE TO READERS: This book has been written and published strictly for informational and educational purposes only. It is not intended to serve as medical advice or to be any form of medical treatment. You should always consult your physician before altering or changing any aspect of your medical treatment and/or undertaking a diet regimen, including the guidelines as described in this book. Do not stop or change any prescription medications without the guidance and advice of your physician. Any use of the information in this book is made on the reader's good judgment after consulting with his or her physician and is the reader's sole responsibility. This book is not intended to diagnose or treat any medical condition and is not a substitute for a physician.

*This book is dedicated to people committed
to making healthy choices!*

CONTENTS

INTRODUCTION
The Importance of Water

"Water doesn't taste good."

"Water's just so boring!"

"I need more flavor with my drinks!"

Everyone KNOWS that drinking water is healthy and necessary, yet many give these excuses as to why they do not drink enough of it. The recipes in this book ensure that water is tasty, flavorful, and most certainly not boring. From simple one- and two-ingredient infusions to fancy sparkling infusions fit for entertaining, these recipes provide countless ways to boost health with antioxidants and lots of water.

BUILDING BLOCK OF THE HUMAN BODY

Leonardo da Vinci once said that "water is the driving force in nature." Just as water is the driving force in nature, it is a foundational building block of the human body and is one of the most important necessities for physical and mental health.

Nearly 70 percent of the human body is composed of water. The brain, bones, organs, and cells require water for the transmission of vital nutrients. As it nourishes our bodies, water aids in digestion, circulates electrolytes and minerals, and assists in detoxification processes. As such, consuming sufficient water on a daily basis is absolutely crucial!

As much as 75 percent of people in this country do not drink enough water and are chronically dehydrated. Dehydration contributes to inflammation in tissues and membranes, and negatively impacts many systems of the body. Skin suffers, leading to premature aging, wrinkles, and discoloration. Digestion suffers, leading to malabsorption and constipation. Brain health suffers, leading to decreased focus and concentration. The muscular system suffers, leading to fatigue, tension, and joint pain. In fact, chronic dehydration can be a major contributing factor to many illnesses, causing headaches, digestive problems, and obesity.

The brain's primary constituent is also water. Adequate hydration is necessary for propagation of chemical messages between the brain and tissues of the body by way of neuronal activity. Several research articles archived in the National Institutes of Health's US National Library of Medicine support that adequate hydration increases concentration, focus, and productivity. As a result, many schools and offices have water readily available for their students and employees.

MAINTAINING HEALTHY WEIGHT

Appropriate water intake helps people maintain a healthy weight and assists with weight loss. People who drink eight or more glasses of water a day eat 200 fewer calories per day than people who drink less. Thirst is often mistaken for hunger, causing people to eat more rather than hydrate more. Drinking water before eating helps not only with hydration, but with overeating, as when thirst is quenched, less food is needed to satiate appetites. Generally, people who drink more water lose more weight and maintain healthier weights than those that drink less water. A study by the American Chemical Society demonstrated that drinking water significantly elevates the resting energy expenditure (REE) in children and adults by up to 25 percent, meaning that more calories are burned at rest in those who drink more water, versus those who drink less. If weight loss is a goal, more water is better!

DAILY WATER RULES

Most people know that drinking lots of water is a healthy habit. However, understanding this concept is different from incorporating it into daily routines! Follow these water rules to increase water intake on a daily basis:

- Drink a large glass of water before every single meal. This helps maintain hydration levels, as well as decreases how much food is eaten during the meal.

- Drink a glass of water within fifteen minutes of waking up in the morning. Put a large glass of water on the nightstand each night and drink it first thing in the morning. Add fresh lemon or lemon essential oil (page 29) to it to encourage detoxification of tissues — see recipes for details!

- Have a pitcher of infused water in the refrigerator at all times. When tasty drinking water is readily available, it is much more likely to be consumed.

- Carry a water bottle at all times. Naturally, people are more likely to drink more water throughout the day if they have it with them! It's convenient to take a water bottle to work, school, the gym, or on the road, and this is an easy way to increase water intake.

- Before snacking, drink a glass of water and wait fifteen minutes. If hunger persists, then have a healthy snack. (An average of 200 calories a day will be spared from your waistline with this simple habit!)

- Swap coffee with tea. Decaffeinated herbal and green teas count as water intake, whereas black tea and coffee do not.

- Make water taste better with fruit, vegetable, and herb infusions. While at restaurants, squeeze lemon, lime, or orange wedges into water, or add essential oils. And at home, sample the numerous infusions found in the recipes section of this book (page 45)!

CHAPTER 1
The Truth about Beverages

Not all drinks are created equal. Many people, even some in the scientific community, believe that chemically flavored water drinks, soft drinks, and energy drinks are acceptable sources of hydration. Although these drinks may have water in them, they do not truly hydrate the body. Even worse, they are filled with fake, and oftentimes toxic, ingredients. Many of these beverages contain preservatives, additives, processed and artificial sugars, dyes, and artificial flavors that are harmful to the body. For example, Coca-Cola has about ten teaspoons of sugar per 12-ounce can. A 12-ounce bottle of Gatorade has approximately five teaspoons of sugar, along with synthetic ingredients. Vitaminwater is no better, with five teaspoons of sugar per 12-ounce serving.

Excessive consumption of sugar has a detrimental effect on health, causing insulin-resistance, diabetes, and weight gain, as well as inflammation that leads to many other degenerative health conditions.

Some use these unhealthy associations with sugar to justify the consumption of artificial sweeteners, like those found in diet and zero-calorie beverages. However, artificial sweeteners are just as unhealthy, if not more so, than regular sugar! Artificial sweeteners also cause insulin-resistance, which can lead to diabetes and obesity. They have also been linked to neurological damage, negatively impacting brain health and function.

Aside from sugars, natural or artificial, there are many other ingredients in these types of beverages that are not particularly healthy. Preservatives, additives, dyes, and artificial flavors have all been associated with a host of mild to extreme health problems, from allergic reactions to carcinogenic status. Generally speaking, these types of ingredients should be avoided, particularly in beverages that are consumed daily.

BENEFITS OF INFUSIONS

Infused waters offer a healthy, delicious alternative to beverages currently found on the market. Combining fruits, vegetables, herbs, spices, and essential oils in water provides crucial hydration to help the body fight inflammation and carry vital nutrients to tissue cells. These types of ingredients contain an abundance of antioxidants, which help to fight free radicals produced by the body that lead to all sorts of health problems, including accelerated aging of cells and tissue. Antioxidants are particularly known for their anti-inflammatory properties.

FRUIT & VEGETABLES

Fruit is always the first thing people think of to use in water infusions because of the delicious flavor enhancement that it offers. Some fruit requires being cut into before adding to infusions, such as lemons and oranges, whereas others can be added whole, like strawberries and blueberries. Cutting up fruit ensures that the yummy, nutritious juices inside it seep into the water and also add to the beauty of the infusions. If you're using a single-serving infusion bottle, fruit can be cut up even more to conserve space.

Vegetables are important to include with infusions because of their power-packed nutrition. While fruit may taste better, veggies pack more nutrition per serving than fruit does. Slicing and dicing veggies is also recommended to make all that nutrition more easily accessible as the water contacts it when making an infusion.

Consuming a diet rich in fruits and vegetables as part of an overall healthy eating plan may reduce the risk of heart attack, stroke, and other forms of heart disease, as well as protect against certain types of cancers. Their fiber also helps reduce the risk of heart disease, as well as the risks of obesity and type II diabetes. Most fruits and vegetables are naturally low in fat, sodium, and calories, and none of them contain cholesterol. Additionally they are sources of many essential nutrients, such as potassium, dietary fiber, vitamin C, and folate. Potassium helps to maintain healthy blood pressure and kidney function. Dietary fiber helps reduce blood cholesterol levels and may lower the risk of heart disease. Vitamin C is important for growing, maintaining, and repairing healthy tissues. Folate helps the body form red blood cells and is particularly important for women that are considering pregnancy and child-bearing.

HERBS & SPICES

Herbs, such as basil and mint, are from plants. Recipes will often call for the leaves of herbs, as with basil leaves or mint leaves, and some will request that the leaves are muddled, or smashed. Muddling the herb leaves breaks them up, freeing up the oils within the leaves to infuse into the water for more flavor and health benefit.

Spices, such as cinnamon and peppercorns, are also from plants, but are from the seeds, berries, barks, or roots of the plant, rather than the leaves. Recipes will often recommend putting spices in a tea ball or sachet so that their flavor and health benefit seeps into the infused water, but that you don't get a mouthful of crunchy spices with each sip!

Studies show that in addition to flavor, herbs and spices offer health benefits such as curbing inflammation because of their high antioxidant count. Tastier drinks are more satisfying than bland ones, and herbs and spices offer flavor boosts without additional calories, fat, sugar, or salt.

ESSENTIAL OILS

Essential oils are natural aromatic compounds found in the seeds, bark, stems, roots, flowers, and other parts of plants. They offer potent smell, flavor, and health benefits to water infusions with just one to two drops. Utilizing oils in the recipes gives a greater health boost to the infusions, as the oils are very concentrated. Using a drop or two of a quality essential oil provides the same medicinal benefit of large quantities of a given fruit or herb. For example, one drop of peppermint essential oil is equivalent to twenty-eight cups of peppermint tea!

Water infusions help create healthy habits for the whole family. Kids love helping to make the infusions, and it is fun to try the various combinations of fruits, veggies, herbs, and essential oils. The possibilities for combining ingredients are really endless, and kids can get very creative!

It is well known that increasing water intake is necessary for dropping excess weight, and fruit, veggie, and herb ingredients can boost that power. Many ingredients increase metabolic activity and promote detoxification in the body, which can assist with weight loss. Replacing other beverages with infused water decreases caloric intake, boosts ability to burn calories at rest, and increases energy levels.

Not only is hydration crucial to brain function, but many of the ingredients for infusions contribute to brain health, too. Powerful phytonutrients found in fruits, veggies, and herbs help to support tissue cells of the brain and body, promoting rejuvenation of body and mind. The powerful combination of ingredients assists in cleansing the detoxification pathways of the body, including the skin, liver, and kidneys. Skin will take on a more youthful appearance, as hydration and antioxidants contribute to slowing down discoloration and the formation of wrinkles.

Water infusions are time- and cost-effective, as well. Infusions can keep for up to three days in the refrigerator; ingredients are inexpensive and you will save money by not purchasing other kinds of costly beverages.

An easy and efficient way to incorporate infused water into daily routines is to use an infusion pitcher or bottle. They're inexpensive and easy to order online, and make creating tasty water infusions even easier! Infusion pitchers and bottles differ from their regular counterparts in that they have a colander-like container down the middle of them, perfectly designed for holding various fruits, veggies, and herbs. Containing ingredients allows for true infusion of the water—the flavors, essences, and nutrients of the ingredients seep into the water, and you don't need to worry about chunks of fruit hitting you in the face each time you take a sip!

Infusion pitchers and bottles make easy recipes even simpler and more convenient. The bottles are great for individual use at home or work, and the pitchers make preparation for weekend picnics or dinner parties a breeze. Depending on the design, a fair amount of fruit, vegetables, and herbs fit into the infusion sleeve, and it's not necessary to adjust the ingredients to refill. Just add more water! Most of the infusion pitchers and bottles are made from plastic that is free of bisphenol-A, or BPA, making it safe for water drinking. (BPA is a synthetic chemical compound that is sometimes used to make some plastics. It has been shown to exhibit hormone-like properties, which has made many people question the safety of consuming food or drinks that have been exposed to it.) Be sure to check the label of your infusion pitcher or bottle to ensure that it is made from plastic that is safe to drink from.

While infusion pitchers are nice for at-home use, infusion bottles are the perfect way to take infused water on the go! There are many inexpensive and attractive travel fruit infusers that are easy to take with you anywhere you go, and the yummy flavors you create will help encourage you to drink more water and not reach for a less healthy option. There are several brands of infusion bottles on the market; look for one that holds at least twenty ounces of water. With this size, more fruit, veggies and herbs will fit into the internal sieve, and it won't be necessary to refill as often.

The recipes in this book have been designed for use with infusion pitchers that hold two liters of water. However, modifying recipes to fit your infuser is super easy. For example, when using an infusion bottle, use just a quarter of the amount of fruit, veggies, and/or herbs noted in the recipe, and fill with water.

CHAPTER 2
The Basics

Top spas around the world have understood and promoted the benefits of infused water for a long time, providing their guests with detoxifying, relaxing, rejuvenating water combinations. Some spas even employ the expertise of a Spa Water Chef, who creates unique water recipes that restore, replenish, and aid relaxation.

With the recipes in this book, think of yourself as your own Spa Water Chef! A trip to the spa is no longer necessary to enjoy the health benefits of nutrient-packed infused water. Making infusions at home allows for control and creativity with your use of ingredients. Water infusions can be simple, with just one ingredient added to water, or complex, with multiple ingredients and steps yielding a flavorful beverage.

INFUSED ICE CUBES

Plain or infused water can be given a boost with infused ice cubes! These cutesy cubes add an adorable element to a party, a brunch, or just a sunny afternoon. These ice cube recipes can complement the infusion recipes or be added to plain still or sparkling water for aesthetics and antioxidant boosts. Infused ice cubes are easy to make and can be stored in the freezer for future use.

The key to making really beautiful, clear ice cubes is to get rid of impurities in the water before pouring into the ice cube trays. First, use filtered water, such as from a Brita (or similar) filter, or from a filtration system connected to the sink. Second, boil the water. Then allow it to cool and boil it again. Boiling the filtered water twice ensures the removal of as many impurities as possible. After pouring this water into ice cube trays and adding infusion ingredients, cover the tray with plastic wrap before freezing. This will ensure that nothing falls into the cubes while they're freezing. While these steps take a bit of time, the result is beautifully clear ice cubes that truly show off the infusion ingredients!

STILL WATER

Most of the water infusion recipes call for still water, or water without bubbles. Still water can come from the sink or tap, but its quality deserves attention. There are often safety concerns with tap water, and many people rely on bottled, spring, filtered, or distilled water to avoid pollutants or impurities.

Having a filtration system in place for tap water is a great way to ensure quality water for the infusion recipes and for drinking in general. Filtration systems can be simple and inexpensive, and can simply consist of a pitcher with a filter like Brita, ZeroWater, or PUR Water. Other filtration systems connect directly to the faucet, so that filtered water comes out. Companies such as Alhambra and Arrowhead sell clean, filtered water in five-gallon bottles that fit on a water cooler, as well as in smaller bottles that can be stored in the refrigerator. Bottom line: Have a source of clean water to ensure the best outcomes for infusion recipes.

SPARKLING WATER

A handful of the recipes in this book call for sparkling water, or water with bubbles. Sparkling water is created by adding carbon dioxide (CO_2) gas to still water. As the gas dissolves in the water, it gives off little bubbles, which is what makes the water sparkle! The sparkling water recipes are especially great for parties and events, as it is a fun way to spruce up plain water.

The easiest way to come by sparkling water is to purchase it from the grocery store. While this is not the most cost-effective option, it is the most convenient. Try to find sparkling water stored in glass bottles, such as San Pellegrino, Perrier, or Gerolsteiner.

Sparkling water can also be made at home, which is more cost-effective than purchasing it. A soda siphon is needed to make it, which requires a metal bottle with a dispenser, a small CO_2

cartridge, and a trigger that injects the gas into the water. Using a soda siphon yields one to two liters of sparkling water, depending on the size of the bottle used. There are commercial options for soda siphons, such as Purefizz, Liss, or SodaStream, available at stores like Target or Bed Bath & Beyond, or online.

QUALITY INGREDIENTS

Quality ingredients make the best water infusions. Most recipes in this book call for fresh fruits, vegetables, or herbs; some call for dried ingredients, and a few call for flowers. It is specifically noted as to which types of ingredients will be best for each recipe.

Always look for organic ingredients when possible. One of the reasons that homemade infusions are so healthy is because they're not filled with preservatives, additives, or fake ingredients. However, much conventional produce is exposed to these types of ingredients during their growth and harvesting. Opting for organic ingredients helps to ensure the purity and quality of the ingredients used for infusions.

Reasonably priced organic produce can be found at farmers' markets, farm co-ops, and some grocery stores. Even Costco and other warehouse stores are now carrying organic produce. Buying what is in season will help keep the cost down, and several recipes have been designed specifically for use during certain times of the year. There are plenty of delicious options to enjoy water infusions all year long.

To prepare your ingredients, be sure to wash fruit, vegetables, and herbs thoroughly to remove dirt, grime, and other impurities from their surfaces. Many recipes call for whole fruits/veggies, or those with the rinds kept on, so it is really important that the ingredients are clean before they are added to the water. This is particularly important if using non-organic ingredients. It is not unusual for the outer surfaces of fresh produce to contain toxins, bacteria, and other contaminants that are not desirable in these water infusions. Also, removing bacteria and other microbes from fresh produce will keep infusions fresh for longer.

The water infusions described in this book are all designed to be made in two-quart pitchers, like those available in stores or online. Glass pitchers are preferred over plastic ones, as plastic can transfer unwanted impurities to the water it is holding. Recipes can be made with built-in compartments for ingredients, but that is not required for them. Once an infusion has been prepared, it can be stored in the refrigerator for two to three days. After that the produce will start to break down and muddy the water a bit. The produce inside will not actually go bad, but the water will not be as attractive and might not taste as good.

ESSENTIAL OILS

Most of the infusion recipes call for a combination of fruits, vegetables, herbs, spices, and occasionally an essential oil or two. Essential oils enhance water infusions with just a couple drops of oil, and just a single drop of oil can change the taste of an infusion dramatically!

However, not all essential oils are created equal, and most essential oils on the market are not safe for internal consumption! As such, we recommend being highly selective when choosing essential oils; look for express indication on the bottle that the oil is safe to consume internally. There are two excellent essential oil companies that offer several oils that are safe to add to water infusions: dōTERRA and Young Living. Their offerings of the oils listed in our recipes are very safe to use internally. However, not all of their oils are designed to be used internally, so be sure to stick to what is listed in the recipes. We cannot stress enough the importance of verifying that an oil is safe to consume! Please read the labels of your oils before adding to your water infusion.

The essential oils from these two companies are carefully distilled or cold pressed from plants that have been harvested from around the world. Specific essential oils have been selected for the recipes in this book. While we encourage you to get creative with the ingredients for infusions, just stick with these essential oils. Below are general descriptions of the oils used in the various recipes and why we like them.

LEMON	Lemon adds a crisp freshness to recipes and is known to help detoxify the body.
LIME	Lime's stimulating and refreshing properties can affect mood and boost immune system function to fight seasonal bugs.
WILD ORANGE	Wild orange impacts mood in a positive way, in that it's uplifting, energizing, and revitalizing. It's great to use in the morning to help wake up and get moving, and smelling this in an infusion is just as powerful as tasting it!
GRAPEFRUIT	Like all the citrus oils, grapefruit is invigorating and uplifting. It also boosts fat-burning as it revs up metabolism.

PEPPERMINT	Peppermint is as potent aromatically as it is in the infusion! It's great for opening airways for improved breathing, as well as for calming an upset stomach and easing headache pain.
LAVENDER	Another potent aromatic, lavender is super calming and relaxing. Recipes with lavender are best suited when winding down for the evening, versus revving up in the morning.

INFUSION TOOLBOX

Most of the recipes in this book are very simple, designed with minimal effort in mind. However, having a few simple tools on hand will make preparation of the infusions faster and easier. Not a requirement for all of the infusions, these tools allow for creating delicious beverages without spending tons of time in the kitchen.

INFUSION PITCHERS & BOTTLES

As described earlier, the absolute easiest way to make these infusions is with a pitcher or bottle that has an infusion sieve inside it. The best combination is a glass pitcher with a stainless steel insert. If that isn't available, then look for BPA-free plastic containers and inserts.

PITCHERS & STIRRING RODS

If you're not using an infusion pitcher, then regulars pitchers and stirring rods are musts! It is recommended to have two to three pitchers in the kitchen so that multiple or big batches of infusions can be made. Glass pitchers are preferred, as plastic can leach impurities into its contents, especially when used with essential oils. Also, glass pitchers will not alter the flavor of infusions as a plastic pitcher may.

Glass stirring rods are encouraged, as well, but are not required. A wooden spoon or spatula can work just as well for these recipes.

MUDDLER

A muddler is what master mixologists and bartenders use to mash ingredients for drinks. Breaking the skin of certain fruits, veggies, and herbs allows for their natural oils to come out, enhancing the smell, flavor, and health benefit of the infusions. Muddlers are simple to use: Place your ingredients on the bottom of a glass or bowl and mash them with the muddler. The mashed ingredients are then ready to use for completion of the recipe. Muddlers can be purchased at stores like Target or Bed Bath & Beyond, and makeshift muddlers can be made from common kitchen utensils like wooden spoons.

FINE-MESH STRAINER OR SIEVE

Strainers and sieves help to keep produce particles out of infusions. Pouring mixtures through the strainer or sieve produces a smooth, easy-to-drink beverage. Certain recipes will specifically call for the use of a strainer or sieve, but feel free to use one in the creation of any recipe.

TEA BALL OR SACHET

A tea ball or sachet comes in handy for a handful of recipes that call for the use of dried herbs and/or flowers. Dried ingredients tend to create lots of little particles, so containing them within a tea ball or sachet allows for infusion of the ingredients without inclusion of all the teeny, tiny bits in the final product. Tea balls are generally stainless steel and come in a variety of sizes. Sachets are very-fine-mesh bags that tie to close. Either one is just fine for recipes that call for their use.

CITRUS JUICER

Sometimes the juice of a fruit is called for, as opposed to the whole or sliced fruit. For these recipes, a citrus juicer comes in very handy. Utilizing a juicer yields a greater amount of juice than simply juicing by hand and allows for collection of juice without pulp or seeds.

BLENDER

Blending certain ingredients allows for the incorporation of a wider variety of ingredients and increases the potency of the infusion. A high-powered blender is recommended for smoothest blending. Running the blended mixture through a fine-mesh sieve will create an even smoother infusion. Blending ingredients also allows for easy absorption of healthy nutrients by the body.

COMMON INGREDIENTS & HEALING PROPERTIES

Flipping through the recipes, certain ingredients pop up time and time again for their potent health benefits or their compatibility with other ingredients. Below are the most commonly used ingredients and their health benefits. Consult this list as you experiment with making your own recipes, so that you can help achieve a certain health goal or find the perfect combination of flavors.

1. LEMON

While its tartness makes the lemon seem extra acidic, it's actually quite alkaline-forming in the body, helping to balance pH of the blood. It's a major detoxifier, known to cleanse the liver, gallbladder, kidneys, and bowels. It contains high levels of vitamin C, a powerful antioxidant that helps prevent the formation of free radicals, thus delaying aging. Lemon has antibacterial properties and helps strengthen blood vessels, thereby helping to lower blood pressure.

DELICIOUS OPTIONS TO INFUSE WITH LEMON: apricots, berries, cherries, cardamom, ginger, nectarines, other citrus fruits, peaches, pears, plums.

2. BASIL

Its high concentration of carotenoids makes basil anti-inflammatory and helpful in protecting cells from free radical damage. Free radical damage can lead to atherosclerosis, asthma, arthritis, heart disease, and stroke, so foods such as basil that are high in carotenoids (and other antioxidants) help decrease the risks of these conditions. Basil is also high in magnesium, which is important for cardiovascular health. The oil found in basil leaves has very strong antibacterial properties, so adding basil essential oil to infusions offers even greater benefit than the leaves alone would.

DELICIOUS OPTIONS TO INFUSE WITH BASIL: apricots, berries, cinnamon, figs, lemons, peaches, pineapple, plums, thyme.

3. MINT

Simply smelling mint activates salivary glands that begin digestion, so it can be very helpful in relieving digestive disorders, particularly nausea and abdominal pain. It also helps with asthma, congestion, and cough by cooling and soothing the nose, throat, and respiratory channels. It can help relieve headaches, depression, and fatigue with its naturally stimulating properties, and has been shown to inhibit the release of histamines that contribute to hay fever and allergies.

DELICIOUS OPTIONS TO INFUSE WITH MINT: apples, berries, cherries, citrus fruits, dates, figs, melons, pears, stone fruits.

4. CUCUMBER

Full of antioxidants, cucumbers are naturally anti-inflammatory and contain many of the same lignans (unique plant polyphenols) that are found in cruciferous veggies such as broccoli and cabbage, and allium veggies such as onions and garlic. Systemic inflammation contributes to many chronic health conditions, such as heart disease, arthritis, autoimmune disorders, and cancer, so decreasing it is imperative for good health.

DELICIOUS OPTIONS TO INFUSE WITH CUCUMBER: berries, citrus fruits, melons, mint.

5. ORANGE

Delicious and nutritious, oranges are a good source of thiamin, folate, and potassium, and a very good source of dietary fiber and vitamin C. The vitamin C helps with maintenance and protection of healthy bones. Beta-carotene protects cells from damage; magnesium helps keep blood pressure in check; folic acid helps with proper brain development; and potassium helps maintain electrolyte balance, as well as a healthy cardiovascular system. Eating oranges has been shown to help reduce mucus, maintain dental health, and balance the ratio of low- and high-density cholesterol.

DELICIOUS OPTIONS TO INFUSE WITH ORANGE: basil, berries, cherries, cilantro, cinnamon, cranberries, figs, ginger, grapes, mint, other citrus fruits, nutmeg, persimmons, pineapple, vanilla.

6. BERRIES

In general, berries .are potent antioxidants and are especially protective against esophageal and colon cancers. They tend to be high in vitamin C and can also contribute calcium, magnesium, folate, and potassium. Not only do they taste great, but the pretty colors of berries also contribute to their superfood status. Berries contain phytochemicals and flavonoids that have been shown to be protective against some forms of cancer. Cranberries and blueberries in particular are helpful in preventing bladder infections. Blueberries and raspberries also contain lutein, which is important for healthy vision. Common varieties include blueberries, raspberries, blackberries, strawberries, cranberries, and red and purple grapes.

DELICIOUS OPTIONS TO INFUSE WITH BERRIES: apples, basil, cardamom, citrus, figs, ginger, lavender, mangos, mint, other berries, peaches, plums, vanilla.

7. GINGER

This versatile herb root holds many a healing property! It is:

- antiviral, antifungal, and antitoxic, which helps it to prevent and treat the common cold

- anti-spastic, which allows it to relieve gas and bloating

- a natural antihistamine, which eases allergies

- anti-inflammatory, which decreases pain and eases nausea induced by seasickness, morning sickness, motion sickness, even that induced by chemotherapy.

Ginger eases coughs and scratchy throats by stimulating the secretion of mucus, which also helps to protect against the development of ulcers. It has been proven to lower cholesterol and help prevent the formation of blood clots, which is key to healthy heart function.

DELICIOUS OPTIONS TO INFUSE WITH GINGER: apricots, apples, berries, citrus fruits, coconut, grapes, passion fruit, peaches, pears, pineapple, plums.

8. CINNAMON STICKS

Adding this warm and comforting spice to your life is an easy way to boost nutrition! Cinnamon is a good source of manganese, fiber, iron, and calcium. It has been shown to help lower LDL (bad) cholesterol, regulate blood sugar, reduce proliferation of leukemia and lymphoma cells, and reduce pain. It has an anti-clotting effect on blood, inhibits bacterial growth and food spoilage, and fights

E. coli. It has been shown to increase sex drive over time and in women, reduce urinary tract infections. Smelling cinnamon boosts cognitive function and memory. And it's delicious!

DELICIOUS OPTIONS TO INFUSE WITH CINNAMON STICKS: apples, citrus fruits, berries, peaches, nectarines.

9. PINEAPPLE

High in vitamin C, pineapple offers great antioxidant value. It helps fight systemic inflammation, which increases blood flow by decreasing blood coagulation, and boosts immune system function to fight colds and other illnesses. It is also high in manganese and thiamin (vitamin B1), both of which support energy production on the cellular level.

DELICIOUS OPTIONS TO INFUSE WITH PINEAPPLE: basil, cilantro, coconut, mangos, papayas.

10. LIME

Like many citrus fruits, limes are full of vitamin C, antioxidants, and flavonoids. These healthy constituents combine to help promote eye health and decrease risk of macular degeneration, boost immune system function to fight colds and fever, promote healthy, clear skin, aid in digestion, and decrease constipation and certain types of arthritis by reducing buildup of uric acid.

DELICIOUS OPTIONS TO INFUSE WITH LIME: apples, berries, cherries, ginger, other citrus fruits, papayas, plums, strawberries.

11. APPLE

Does an apple a day really keep the doctor away? It appears so, with all of the amazing health benefits that this tasty fruit packs! A good source of dietary fiber and vitamin C, apples also contain antioxidant flavonoids, which have been shown to help prevent and treat a variety of conditions. One flavonoid, phloridzin, is found only in apples, and may increase bone density and help prevent osteoporosis in post-menopausal women. Apples also contain boron, which helps strengthen bones. Quercetin, another flavonoid, has been shown to protect brain cells from the free radical damage that leads to Alzheimer's. The pectin in apples is thought to lower bad (LDL) cholesterol and help with diabetes management. The flavonoids and other properties found in apples have been shown to be instrumental in the prevention of lung, breast, colon, and liver cancers.

DELICIOUS OPTIONS TO INFUSE WITH APPLES: cardamom, cinnamon, cranberries, currants, ginger, mangos, oranges, rosemary.

12. GRAPE

Crisp and crunchy grapes pack a lot of punch with their vast array of antioxidants, vitamins, and minerals. In addition to containing vitamins A and C, grapes boast vitamin B6 (known to help people with morning sickness, Parkinson's disease, heart disease, and autism) and folate (most notable for its role in helping/preventing heart disease, stroke, and cancer, but also known for helping with obesity, depression, schizophrenia, rheumatoid arthritis, fertility, kidney disease, macular degeneration, bone health, and menopause). Grapes also contain the essential minerals potassium, calcium, iron, phosphorus, magnesium, and selenium. This rockin' combination of vitamins and minerals work together to help grapes improve and/or prevent the following: asthma, heart disease, migraines, constipation, indigestion, fatigue, kidney disorders, Alzheimer's, breast cancer, macular degeneration, cataracts, cholesterol, and bacterial and viral infections.

DELICIOUS OPTIONS TO INFUSE WITH GRAPES: citrus fruits, ginger, raisins.

13. POMEGRANATE

This beautiful fruit and its juice are full of antioxidant flavonoids that counteract cancer-causing free radicals and help support normal blood flow to the heart, helping to avoid heart disease and stroke. It is a good source of vitamins A, C, and E, and the mineral folate. It helps maintain clear, youthful skin by keeping blood platelets together. The combination of antioxidants, vitamins, and minerals makes it a prime candidate to assist in preventing many types of cancer and heart disease, as well as helping with numerous chronic and degenerative conditions.

DELICIOUS OPTIONS TO INFUSE WITH POMEGRANATE: apples, citrus fruits, cucumbers, mint, tropical fruits.

14. KIWI

The many flavonoids, vitamins, and minerals of kiwis make them an excellent source of antioxidants and overall nutrition. Kiwis have been shown to be particularly helpful with respiratory problems in children, notably decreasing symptoms of asthma, shortness of breath, nighttime coughing, wheezing, chronic coughing, and runny nose. It's important to note that these results are not traceable to just the content of vitamin C or potassium, but to substances which are still largely unknown, but are contained within kiwi fruit. (Once again, whole foods are greater than the sum of their parts!) This combination of nutrition in kiwis helps protect DNA from mutations, and their high fiber content helps prevent colon cancer.

DELICIOUS OPTIONS TO INFUSE WITH KIWI: apples, berries, cherries, citrus fruits, coconut, mangos.

15. PEACH

Peaches are full of antioxidants, including vitamins A and C. Vitamin A helps improve eye health, decreasing risk of macular degeneration, and vitamin C helps improve skin texture and health. As such, peach is often a key ingredient in skin moisturizers. Peaches, and other stone fruit, have also been shown to decrease the effects of diabetes, metabolic syndrome, and cardiovascular disease.

DELICIOUS OPTIONS TO INFUSE WITH PEACH: berries, cinnamon, citrus, ginger, other stone fruits, vanilla.

16. BLUEBERRY

One of the highest concentrations of antioxidants are found in blueberries, specifically compounds that improve the health of the tissues that make up the brain and nervous system. Blueberries help lower blood pressure and decrease the oxidation of cholesterol, which is what leads to clogging of arteries and blood vessels. They also help regulate blood sugar, as well as improve cognitive function.

DELICIOUS OPTIONS TO INFUSE WITH BLUEBERRY: berries, cardamom, figs, ginger, lavender, lemons, mangos.

17. GRAPEFRUIT

High in vitamin C, grapefruit is a major immune system booster. It's a cold fighter, helping to prevent and decrease the symptoms of colds when they come on. Since vitamin C is an antioxidant, grapefruit helps prevent the formation of free radicals, which assists in stopping the cascade that leads to inflammation. Grapefruit is a great liver detoxifier, helping the body excrete toxic compounds. It also boosts metabolic activity, assisting in fat burning.

DELICIOUS OPTIONS TO INFUSE WITH GRAPEFRUIT: basil, citrus fruits, mint, rosemary, thyme, vanilla.

18. ROSEMARY

This hearty herb contains compounds that most notably stimulate and protect brain functions. It has been shown to improve memory, focus, and concentration by increasing blood flow to the head and brain. It also fights free radical formation and damage, and helps to delay premature aging of the brain. It also supports immune system function and improves digestion.

DELICIOUS OPTIONS TO INFUSE WITH ROSEMARY: apples, apricots, citrus fruits, currants, grapes, pears.

19. LAVENDER

Relaxing lavender is most noted for its tension-relieving and sleep-promoting properties. It also helps many systems of the body. It is a natural bug repellent, helps heal acne, eases muscle tension and soreness, stimulates urine flow and increases or promotes respiratory function. It promotes the production of gastric juices, which can aid in digestion, and has antibacterial properties that enhance immune system function.

DELICIOUS OPTIONS TO INFUSE WITH LAVENDER: blueberries, blackberries, lemons, peaches, raspberries.

20. MELON

All melons are high in vitamins A and C, and potassium. As such, they decrease systemic inflammation, which helps every system of the body. They also help boost immune system function to fight colds and circulatory function to lower blood pressure.

DELICIOUS OPTIONS TO INFUSE WITH MELON: berries, citrus fruits, cucumbers, lemongrass, lemons, mint.

CHAPTER 3
Recipes

The recipes in this book vary from very simple to complex. We'll begin with simple fruit infusions, advancing to vegetable, herb, and mixed-flavor combinations. Some recipes list specific health benefits with their consumption, while others are designed for enjoyment during specific times of the year. The final section includes recipes for specific health goals, such as post-workout, stress-relieving, and circulation-improving combinations. Use them as a guideline, but feel free to substitute ingredients or add your own twist.

Our goal with the recipes is to combine flavors to produce delicious and, more often than not, naturally sweet beverages. If you feel that you absolutely have to sweeten an infusion, then you may use a tiny amount of stevia (liquid or granular). It is the most accepted, least harmful sugar substitute. A teeny amount of honey or maple syrup would also be acceptable. (Do not, under any circumstances, add any other sugar or artificial sweetener! You will be doing yourself a huge disservice.)

FRUIT & VEGGIE INFUSIONS

Infusion recipes can be as basic as adding one type of fruit to water. As such, our recipes start simplistic, with just a couple of fruit and vegetable ingredients added to water, and get more complex throughout the book. Keep in mind that fruit ingredients are pretty easy to swap. For example, if you're not a fan of lemon, feel free to use lime, orange, or grapefruit instead.

STRAWBERRY LEMON

1 cup strawberries, whole
½ cup strawberries, hulled and sliced
1 lemon, sliced into wheels
ice
1½ quarts still water

Add fruit to the insert of a 2-quart infusion pitcher. Add desired amount of ice to pitcher, then fill with water. Allow to steep for at least 30 minutes, but preferably for 2 to 3 hours, before serving.

TIP: We like slicing citrus into wheels because it looks so pretty! But as long as it's cut up to allow the juices and goodness to seep out of it, it doesn't really matter how it's cut.

STRAWBERRY PEACH

1 cup strawberries, whole
½ cup strawberries, hulled and sliced
1 peach, pitted and sliced
ice
1½ quarts still water

Add fruit to the insert of a 2-quart infusion pitcher. Add desired amount of ice to pitcher, then fill with water. Allow to steep for at least 30 minutes, but preferably for 2 to 3 hours, before serving.

TIP: This recipe is really beautiful, with some sliced berries and some whole! But if you're in a hurry, you can just throw the whole berries in there without slicing first.

BLUEBERRY LEMON

1½ cups blueberries
2 lemons, sliced into wheels
ice
1½ quarts still water

Add fruit to the insert of a 2-quart infusion pitcher. Add desired amount of ice to pitcher, then fill with water. Allow to steep for at least 30 minutes, but preferably for 2 to 3 hours, before serving.

TIP: Between the invigorating lemon and brain-boosting blueberries, this combo is perfect for an afternoon pick-me-up!

PINEAPPLE STRAWBERRY

1½ cups pineapple, hulled and cut into chunks
1 cup strawberries, hulled and sliced
ice
1½ quarts still water

Add fruit to the insert of a 2-quart infusion pitcher. Add desired amount of ice to pitcher, then fill with water. Allow to steep for at least 30 minutes, but preferably for 2 to 3 hours, before serving.

TIP: If you don't have an infusion pitcher, just layer the fruit along the bottom of a 2-quart pitcher!

RASPBERRY NECTARINE

1 cup raspberries
2 nectarines, pitted and sliced
ice
1½ quarts still water

Add fruit to the insert of a 2-quart infusion pitcher. Add desired amount of ice to pitcher, then fill with water. Allow to steep for at least 30 minutes, but preferably for 2 to 3 hours, before serving.

TIP: Raspberries have teeny tiny seeds that can be aggravating to teeth and gums, so this recipe is better off made with an infusion pitcher, rather than a regular pitcher.

LEMON CUCUMBER

2 lemons, sliced into wheels
1 small cucumber, sliced into rounds
ice
1½ quarts still water

Add fruit to the insert of a 2-quart infusion pitcher. Add desired amount of ice to pitcher, then fill with water. Allow to steep for at least 30 minutes, but preferably for 2 to 3 hours, before serving.

TIP: Like lemons, cucumbers are extremely detoxifying. This combo is great for post-workout refreshment!

SPICY LEMON
(LEMON JALAPEÑO)

1½ lemons, sliced into wheels
Juice of 1 lemon
½ jalapeño, seeded and sliced into wheels
ice
1½ quarts still water

Add lemon and jalapeño to the insert of a 2-quart infusion pitcher. Add desired amount of ice to pitcher, then fill with water. Allow to steep for at least 30 minutes, but preferably for 2 to 3 hours, before serving.

TIP: Want your infusion super spicy? Leave the seeds in! It's the seeds that determine the spice level of the pepper, so leaving them in will boost your spice quotient by quite a bit.

"BLOODY MARY" (CELERY TOMATO PEPPERCORN)

2 large celery stalks, cut into 3-inch pieces
1 tomato, seeded and cut into wedges
juice of 1 lemon
1 tablespoon black peppercorns
ice
1½ quarts still water

Add celery, tomato, and lemon juice to the insert of a 2-quart infusion pitcher. Place peppercorns in a tea ball or sachet and add to the insert. Add desired amount of ice to pitcher, then fill with water. Allow to steep for at least 30 minutes, but preferably for 2 to 3 hours, before serving. Remove tea ball or sachet before serving.

TIP: This combo is wonderful with Sunday brunch or taco night!

PINEAPPLE CUCUMBER MINT

1½ cups pineapple, hulled and cut into chunks
1 small cucumber, sliced into rounds
2 to 4 sprigs fresh mint
ice
1½ quarts still water

Add pineapple, cucumber, and mint to the insert of a 2-quart infusion pitcher. Add desired amount of ice to pitcher, then fill with water. Allow to steep for at least 30 minutes, but preferably for 2 to 3 hours, before serving.

TIP: This is a gorgeous combo for an afternoon picnic—serve in tumblers over ice garnished with a chunk of pineapple and sprig of mint on the side of the glass.

STRAWBERRY CUCUMBER

1 cup strawberries, whole
½ cup strawberries, hulled and sliced
1 small cucumber, sliced into rounds
ice
1½ quarts still water

Add strawberries and cucumber to the insert of a 2-quart infusion pitcher. Add desired amount of ice to pitcher, then fill with water. Allow to steep for at least 30 minutes, but preferably for 2 to 3 hours, before serving.

TIP: The size of inserts in infusion pitchers will vary, so alternate adding ingredients so that you don't end up with too much of one thing!

HERBAL INFUSIONS

Adding herbs to infusions provides an opportunity for very interesting flavor combinations, not to mention increasing the antioxidant value of the beverages you create. Most recipes that call for the leaves of herb plants also recommend muddling, or smashing, those leaves to enhance the flavor infused into the water. As for spices, it's always a good idea to put them in a tea ball or sachet, even if using an infusion pitcher, to avoid floaties in your water.

STRAWBERRY BASIL

1 cup strawberries, whole
½ cup strawberries, hulled and sliced
2 to 4 sprigs fresh basil
ice
1½ quarts still water

Add strawberries and basil to the insert of a 2-quart infusion pitcher. Add desired amount of ice to pitcher, then fill with water. Allow to steep for at least 30 minutes, but preferably for 2 to 3 hours, before serving.

TIP: Breaking up the basil leaves just a bit before adding them to the infuser insert will leach even more basil flavor into your infusion!

CUCUMBER BASIL

1 small cucumber, sliced into rounds
2 to 4 sprigs fresh basil
ice
1½ quarts still water

Add cucumber and basil to the insert of a 2-quart infusion pitcher. Add desired amount of ice to pitcher, then fill with water. Allow to steep for at least 30 minutes, but preferably for 2 to 3 hours, before serving.

TIP: This is one of the more savory recipes in the book and goes very well with spicy meals, such as Indian or Thai food.

ORANGE SAGE

1½ oranges, sliced into wheels
juice of ½ orange
10 to 12 leaves fresh sage
ice
1½ quarts still water

Add orange, orange juice, and sage to the insert of a 2-quart infusion pitcher. Add desired amount of ice to pitcher, then fill with water. Allow to steep for at least 30 minutes, but preferably for 2 to 3 hours, before serving.

TIP: Occasionally we recommend adding fresh-squeezed fruit juice to the infusion for that much more flavor!

BLUEBERRY SAGE

2 cups blueberries
10 to 12 leaves fresh sage
ice
1½ quarts still water

Scrunch up the sage a bit, then add it with the blueberries to the insert of a 2-quart infusion pitcher. Add desired amount of ice to pitcher, then fill with water. Allow to steep for at least 30 minutes, but preferably for 2 to 3 hours, before serving

TIP: Scrunching, or muddling, the sage before adding it helps to break up the herb, releasing its natural nutrition and taste.

LIME VANILLA

1 lime, sliced into rounds
juice of 1 lime
1 medium vanilla bean, sliced lengthwise
ice
1½ quarts still water

Add lime, lime juice, and vanilla bean to the insert of a 2-quart infusion pitcher. Add desired amount of ice to pitcher, then fill with water. Allow to steep for at least 30 minutes, but preferably for 2 to 3 hours, before serving.

TIP: Adding vanilla bean to infusions produces an almost creamy quality to the beverage, delicious on a cool morning or evening by the fire.

ORANGE JUNIPER

1½ oranges, sliced into wheels
juice of ½ orange
2 tablespoons fresh juniper berries
ice
1½ quarts still water

Add oranges and orange juice to the insert of a 2-quart infusion pitcher. Place juniper berries in a tea ball or sachet and add to insert. Add desired amount of ice to pitcher, then fill with water. Allow to steep for at least 30 minutes, but preferably for 2 to 3 hours, before serving. Remove tea ball or sachet before serving.

TIP: Juniper berries provide a very strong flavor, so you may want to remove the tea ball or sachet with them in it after 30 minutes or steeping, even if you let the rest steep longer.

WATERMELON ROSEMARY

2 cups watermelon, cubed
2 to 4 sprigs fresh rosemary
ice
1½ quarts still water

Add watermelon and rosemary to the insert of a 2-quart infusion pitcher. Add desired amount of ice to pitcher, then fill with water. Allow to steep for at least 30 minutes, but preferably for 2 to 3 hours, before serving.

TIP: Using an infusion pitcher is especially useful when making an infusion with these two ingredients, so that you get nice, smooth, delicious water, without having to worry about seeds, stems, or other floaties in your drink!

RASPBERRY MINT

2 cups raspberries, divided
4 sprigs fresh mint, divided
ice
1½ quarts still water

In a glass or bowl, combine 1 cup of the raspberries and 2
sprigs of mint and mash with a muddler, working to break
up the mint leaves. Pour mixture into the insert of a 2-quart
infusion pitcher and add remaining raspberries and mint. Add
desired amount of ice to pitcher, then fill with water. Allow to
steep for at least 30 minutes, but preferably for 2 to 3 hours,
before serving.

TIP: Sometimes particles of fruit, veggies, herbs, or spices end
up in the water, even when using an infusion pitcher. If this
happens, just pour the mixture through a fine-mesh sieve
to strain out particles before serving.

LEMON MINT

2 lemons, sliced into wheels
2 to 4 sprigs fresh mint
ice
1½ quarts still water

Add lemons and mint to the insert of a 2-quart infusion pitcher. Add desired amount of ice to pitcher, then fill with water. Allow to steep for at least 30 minutes, but preferably for 2 to 3 hours, before serving.

TIP: This classic combination makes a delicious summer "mocktail" — just replace the still water with sparkling water!

PEAR FENNEL

2 pears, cored and cut into chunks
½ bulb fennel, shaved
ice
1½ quarts still water

Layer fruit and fennel along the bottom of a 2-quart pitcher.
Cover with desired amount of ice, then fill with water. Allow to
steep for at least 30 minutes, but preferably for 2 to 3 hours,
before serving.

TIP: Not sure what fennel looks like? It has a white or light
green bulb, with a stalk and feathery green leaves. You can
"shave" it using a mandolin, cheese slicer, or knife.

LEMON LAVENDER

1½ lemons, sliced into wheels
2 sprigs fresh lavender
juice of ½ lemon
1 drop lavender essential oil
ice
1½ quarts still water

Add lemons and fresh lavender to the insert of a 2-quart infusion pitcher, then add lemon juice and essential oil. Add desired amount of ice to pitcher, then fill with water. Allow to steep for at least 30 minutes, but preferably for 2 to 3 hours, before serving.

TIP: Just a reminder: Not all essential oils are created equal, and most are not safe for internal consumption! Essential oils from Young Living and dōTERRA are approved for internal use.

LIME GINGER

2 limes, sliced into wheels
3-inch piece of fresh ginger, peeled and sliced
1 drop lime essential oil
ice
1½ quarts still water

Add limes and ginger to the insert of a 2-quart infusion pitcher, then add essential oil. Add desired amount of ice to pitcher, then fill with water. Allow to steep for at least 30 minutes, but preferably for 2 to 3 hours, before serving.

TIP: Ginger helps boost fat-burning in the body by boosting metabolism, while lime is an excellent detoxifier. As such, this combo is great for people looking to drop some weight!

PARSLEY MINT

1 small handful fresh parsley, stems and leaves
2 to 4 sprigs fresh mint
ice
1½ quarts still water

Add parsley and mint to the insert of a 2-quart infusion pitcher. Add desired amount of ice to pitcher, then fill with water. Allow to steep for at least 30 minutes, but preferably for 2 to 3 hours, before serving.

TIP: Parsley is an excellent palate cleanser, so this combo is great to serve between courses at a dinner party.

FANCY INFUSIONS

Once you start experimenting with water infusions, you'll see how easy it is to modify recipes and combine flavors. That's how we came up with our fancy infusions! These recipes have three or more ingredients each, bringing together different fruits complemented by various herbs and spices. When layering ingredients in the infusion pitchers, keep in mind that the size of the internal sieve may vary pitcher to pitcher. Just layer the ingredients, instead of adding all of one then all of the next. That way you'll always get a balanced infusion, even if you don't end up needing all of the ingredients. As always, feel free to play with flavor profiles by adding and removing different fruits and herbs.

PEAR RASPBERRY ROSEMARY

1 crisp pear, cored and cut into chunks
1 cup raspberries
2 to 4 sprigs fresh rosemary
ice
1½ quarts still water

Add pear, raspberries, and rosemary to the insert of a 2-quart infusion pitcher. Add desired amount of ice to pitcher, then fill with water. Allow to steep for at least 30 minutes, but preferably for 2 to 3 hours, before serving.

TIP: Rosemary is an amazing complement to meat dishes, so this combo is an excellent pairing to lamb, pork, or chicken dinners.

ORANGE LEMON CILANTRO

1 orange, sliced into wheels
1 lemon, sliced into wheels
1 small bunch fresh cilantro, stems and leaves
1 drop orange essential oil
ice
1½ quarts still water

Add oranges, lemons, and cilantro to the insert of a 2-quart infusion pitcher, then add the essential oil. Add desired amount of ice to pitcher, then fill with water. Allow to steep for at least 30 minutes, but preferably for 2 to 3 hours, before serving.

TIP: Cilantro is a common ingredient in Latin cooking, so the hint of the herb in this combo makes this an ideal beverage choice with tacos, enchiladas, or other Mexican dishes.

CHERRY LIME VANILLA

2 cups cherries, pitted and halved
1½ limes, sliced into wheels
1 medium vanilla bean, sliced lengthwise
ice
juice of ½ lime
1½ quarts still water

Add cherries, limes, and vanilla bean to the insert of a 2-quart infusion pitcher. Add desired amount of ice to pitcher, then add lime juice and fill with water. Allow to steep for at least 30 minutes, but preferably for 2 to 3 hours, before serving.

TIP: Make a delicious and healthy "soda" by swapping still water in this recipe for sparkling.

STRAWBERRY CUCUMBER BASIL

½ cup strawberries, hulled and sliced
4 sprigs fresh basil, divided
1 cup strawberries, whole
1 small cucumber, sliced into rounds
ice
1½ quarts still water

In a glass or bowl, combine sliced strawberries and the leaves of 2 sprigs of fresh basil and mash with a muddler, working to break the basil leaves. Pour mixture into the insert of a 2-quart infusion pitcher, then add whole strawberries, cucumbers, and remaining basil.

TIP: Add desired amount of ice to pitcher, then fill with water. Allow to steep for at least 30 minutes, but preferably for 2 to 3 hours, before serving.

BLUEBERRY LEMON MINT

2 cups blueberries, divided
juice of ½ lemon
1½ lemons, sliced into wheels
4 sprigs fresh mint, divided
ice
1½ quarts still water

In a glass or bowl, combine ½ cup blueberries, lemon juice, and the leaves of 2 sprigs of fresh mint and mash with a muddler, working to break the mint leaves. Pour mixture into the insert of a 2-quart infusion pitcher, then add remaining blueberries, lemons, and mint.

Add desired amount of ice to pitcher, then fill with water. Allow to steep for at least 30 minutes, but preferably for 2 to 3 hours, before serving.

TIP: Sometimes muddling ingredients causes particles to leak out from the sieve insert into the water. To get rid of these floaties, just pour the water mixture through a fine-mesh sieve before serving.

LEMON GINGER MINT

2 lemons, sliced into wheels
3-inch piece of fresh ginger, peeled and sliced
4 sprigs fresh mint
1 drop lemon essential oil
ice
1½ quarts still water

Add lemons, ginger, and mint to the insert of a 2-quart infusion pitcher, then add essential oil. Add desired amount of ice to pitcher, then fill with water. Allow to steep for at least 30 minutes, but preferably for 2 to 3 hours, before serving.

TIP: This combination is an amazing weight loss aid, as lemon detoxifies the system, encouraging metabolism, and ginger and mint both boost metabolic activity! This metabolic boost leads to faster calorie and fat burning, and ultimately weight loss.

PEACH CHERRY MINT

1 cup cherries, pitted and halved, divided
4 sprigs fresh mint, divided
2 peaches, pitted and sliced
ice
1½ quarts still water

In a glass or bowl, combine ½ cup cherries and the leaves of 2 sprigs of fresh mint and mash with a muddler, working to break up the mint leaves. Pour mixture into the insert of a 2-quart infusion pitcher, then add peaches, remaining cherries, and remaining mint.

Add desired amount of ice to pitcher, then fill with water. Allow to steep for at least 30 minutes, but preferably for 2 to 3 hours, before serving.

TIP: Stone fruit, like peaches and cherries, are most plentiful during the summer months. Cut up stone fruit and freeze it, and you'll have ingredients on hand for this beverage all year round!

PINEAPPLE ORANGE VANILLA

2 cups pineapple, hulled and cubed
1 orange, sliced into wheels
1 medium vanilla bean, sliced lengthwise
1 drop orange essential oil
ice
1½ quarts still water

Add pineapple, oranges, and vanilla bean to the insert of a 2-quart infusion pitcher, then add essential oil. Add desired amount of ice to pitcher, then fill with water. Allow to steep for at least 30 minutes, but preferably for 2 to 3 hours, before serving.

TIP: The addition of vanilla bean to this infusion makes this tropical fruit sensation taste like a Creamsicle!

ORANGE VANILLA CINNAMON

1½ oranges, sliced into wheels
2 medium vanilla beans, sliced lengthwise
2 cinnamon sticks
juice of ½ orange
1 drop orange essential oil
ice
1½ quarts still water

Add oranges, vanilla beans, and cinnamon sticks to the insert of a 2-quart infusion pitcher. Add desired amount of ice to pitcher, add orange juice and essential oil, then fill with water. Allow to steep for at least 30 minutes, but preferably for 2 to 3 hours, before serving.

TIP: Make this combo without ice, or even with hot water, for a comforting tea-like beverage.

APPLE CINNAMON GINGER

2 crisp apples, cored and sliced
2 cinnamon sticks
3-inch piece of fresh ginger, peeled and sliced
ice
1½ quarts still water

Add apples, cinnamon sticks, and ginger to the insert of a
2-quart infusion pitcher. Add desired amount of ice to pitcher,
then fill with water. Allow to steep for at least 30 minutes, but
preferably for 2 to 3 hours, before serving.

TIP: Served warm, this yummy combo resembles apple cider!

APRICOT CHERRY VANILLA

2 apricots, pitted and sliced
2 cups cherries, pitted and halved
1 medium vanilla bean, sliced lengthwise
ice
1½ quarts still water

Add apricots, cherries, and vanilla bean to the insert of a 2-quart infusion pitcher. Add desired amount of ice to pitcher, then fill with water. Allow to steep for at least 30 minutes, but preferably for 2 to 3 hours, before serving.

TIP: This combo makes a delicious healthy soda, too—just swap the still water for sparkling water.

ORANGE MINT VANILLA

1½ oranges, sliced into wheels
4 sprigs fresh mint
1 medium vanilla bean, sliced lengthwise
juice of ½ orange
1 drop orange essential oil
ice
1½ quarts still water

Add oranges, mint, and vanilla bean to the insert of a 2-quart infusion pitcher. Add desired amount of ice to pitcher, then add orange juice and essential oil, and fill with water. Allow to steep for at least 30 minutes, but preferably for 2 to 3 hours, before serving.

TIP: Mint and orange together are an uplifting combo, making this recipe a great option for a healthy jumpstart to your day.

PINEAPPLE CUCUMBER PARSLEY

2 cups pineapple, hulled and cubed
1 small cucumber, sliced into rounds
1 small bunch fresh parsley, stems and leaves
ice
1½ quarts still water

Add pineapple, cucumber, and parsley to the insert of a 2-quart infusion pitcher. Add desired amount of ice to pitcher, then fill with water. Allow to steep for at least 30 minutes, but preferably for 2 to 3 hours, before serving.

TIP: Parsley is a wonderful palate cleanser, so this combo would be a great addition to serve between courses at a dinner party!

PEACH PLUM SAGE

2 peaches, pitted and sliced
2 plums, pitted and sliced
10 to 12 leaves fresh sage
ice
1½ quarts still water

Add peaches, plums, and sage to the insert of a 2-quart infusion pitcher. Add desired amount of ice to pitcher, then fill with water. Allow to steep for at least 30 minutes, but preferably for 2 to 3 hours, before serving.

TIP: Sage is classically combined with butter in cooking and is often an amazing complement to pasta dishes. This beverage would go perfectly with such a meal.

PINEAPPLE STRAWBERRY MINT

½ cup strawberries, hulled and sliced
4 sprigs fresh mint, divided
2 cups pineapple, hulled and cubed
1 cup strawberries, whole
ice
1½ quarts still water

In a glass or bowl, combine sliced strawberries and the leaves from 2 sprigs of mint and mash with a muddler, working to break up the mint leaves. Pour mixture into the insert of a 2-quart infusion pitcher, then add pineapple, whole strawberries, and remaining mint.

Add desired amount of ice to pitcher, then fill with water. Allow to steep for at least 30 minutes, but preferably for 2 to 3 hours, before serving. Pour mixture through a fine-mesh sieve to strain out particles before serving.

TIP: This combo makes an excellent "mocktail"—simply swap the still water for sparkling!

PEACH MANGO MINT

1 mango, pitted and cubed, divided
4 sprigs fresh mint, divided
2 peaches, pitted and sliced
ice
1½ quarts still water

In a glass or bowl, combine half the mango and the leaves from 2 sprigs of mint and mash with a muddler, working to break up the mint leaves. Pour mixture into the insert of a 2-quart insertion pitcher, then add peaches, remaining mango, and remaining mint.

Add desired amount of ice to pitcher, then fill with water. Allow to steep for at least 30 minutes, but preferably for 2 to 3 hours, before serving. Pour mixture through a fine-mesh sieve to strain out particles before serving.

TIP: This tropical-inspired beverage pairs well with chicken or fish dishes.

LEMON ORANGE JUNIPER

2 tablespoons fresh juniper berries
1½ lemons, sliced into wheels
juice of ½ lemon
1½ oranges, sliced into wheels
juice of ½ orange
1 drop lemon essential oil
1 drop orange essential oil
ice
1½ quarts still water

Place juniper berries in a tea ball or sachet, then add it, plus the lemons and oranges, to the insert of a 2-quart infusion pitcher. Add desired amount of ice to pitcher. Add essential oils, lemon juice, and orange juice, then fill with water. Allow to steep for at least 30 minutes, but preferably for 2 to 3 hours, before serving. Remove tea ball or sachet after 30 minutes, regardless of how long the rest of the mixture steeps.

TIP: Earthy juniper berries combine with zesty citrus to provide a refreshing and invigorating beverage.

CUCUMBER-MINT-CILANTRO WATERMELON COOLER

½ cup cucumber, sliced into rounds
1 cup watermelon, cut into 1-inch chunks
1 sprig fresh mint
1 sprig fresh cilantro
2 quarts still water

Add cucumber, watermelon, mint, and cilantro to the insert of a 2-quart infusion pitcher. Add desired amount of ice to pitcher, then fill with water. Allow to steep for at least 30 minutes, but preferably for 2 to 3 hours, before serving.

TIP: This mixture is the perfect accompaniment to a summer barbecue.

TROPICAL VACATION ESCAPE

1 lime, sliced into wheels
1 cup star fruit, peeled and sliced into "stars"
1 orange, sliced into wheels
2 kiwis, peeled and sliced into wheels
6 to 8 sprigs fresh cilantro
ice
1½ quarts still water

Add limes, star fruit, oranges, kiwis, and cilantro to the insert of a 2-quart infusion pitcher. Add desired amount of ice to pitcher, then fill with water. Allow to steep for at least 30 minutes, but preferably for 2 to 3 hours, before serving.

TIP: The formal name for star fruit is carambola, and its taste has been described as a mixture of apple, pear, grape, and citrus. Its skin is waxy, but is okay to eat. We recommend cutting the star fruit on its short axis to take advantage of its unique star shape!

STAR BURST

1 cup strawberries, hulled and sliced
1 orange, sliced into wheels
1 grapefruit, sliced into wheels
1 medium vanilla bean, sliced lengthwise
ice
2 drops lemon essential oil
1½ quarts still water

Add strawberries, oranges, grapefruit, and vanilla bean to the insert of a 2-quart infusion pitcher. Add desired amount of ice to pitcher, add the essential oil, then fill with water. Allow to steep for at least 30 minutes, but preferably for 2 to 3 hours, before serving.

TIP: Consider serving over Citrus Burst Ice Cubes (page 144) for some extra bliss!

CHERRY MOJITO SPLASH

1½ cups cherries, pitted and halved
juice of 2 limes
2 dates, pitted and halved
10 to 12 fresh mint leaves
1 cup still water
1½ quarts sparkling water

Add cherries, lime juice, dates, mint, and the 1 cup of still water to a blender and blend until smooth, approximately 1 minute. Pour through a fine-mesh sieve into a 2-quart pitcher. Add lime halves to the insert of 2-quart infusion pitcher, then fill pitcher with sparkling water. Serve immediately, or refrigerate infusion for 1 to 2 hours before serving to further intensify flavors.

TIP: Blending ingredients allows for greater mixture of water with the ingredients for an infusion, which heightens the infusion's nutritional value.

RUBY RED RAZZMATAZZ SPARKLER

2 cups raspberries
1 cup cherries, pitted and halved
½ cup pomegranate seeds
1 teaspoon lemon juice
2 drops lemon essential oil
1½ quarts sparkling water

Add raspberries, cherries, and pomegranate seeds to the insert of a 2-quart infusion pitcher. Add desired amount of ice to pitcher, add the lemon juice and essential oil, then fill with water. Allow to steep for at least 30 minutes, but preferably for 2 to 3 hours, before serving.

TIP: By halving the cherries before adding to the insert, your infusion will turn a beautiful pinkish shade, and the color will deepen the longer the fruit infuses!

SPARKLING DELIGHT

1 cup strawberries, hulled
2 peaches, pitted and halved
1 teaspoon lemon juice
2 drops orange essential oil
1½ quarts sparkling water

Add the strawberries and peaches to blender and blend until smooth, approximately 1 minute. Pour mixture through a fine-mesh strainer into a 2-quart pitcher, then add lemon juice, essential oil, and sparkling water. Chill infusion for 2 hours before serving. Consider serving over Nectarine and Basil Ice Cubes (page 142) for more summer fruit fun!

TIP: We recommend using a regular pitcher for this recipe, since the fruit ingredients are blended before adding to water. However, you could easily modify the recipe to use an infusion pitcher—just put the fruit directly in the infusion insert without blending.

BLUEBERRY LEMONADE SPARKLE

1 cup blueberries
juice of 1 lemon
2 dates, pitted and halved
1 cup still water
1 lemon, sliced into wheels
1½ quarts sparkling water

Add blueberries, lemon juice, dates, and the 1 cup of still water to a blender and blend until smooth, approximately 1 minute. Pour mixture through a fine-mesh strainer into the base of a 2-quart infusion pitcher, add the lemon slices to the insert, then add sparkling water to the pitcher. Chill infusion for 2 hours before serving.

TIP: Adding dates to the blended mixture creates the sweetness necessary to call this "lemonade." So if you find that you prefer a sweeter infusion, consider blending dates with water to add to other infusions, too.

SEASONAL INFUSIONS

One of the best ways to increase the cost-effectiveness of making your own water infusions is to use fruit that is in season. The following recipes all use ingredients that are most readily available during certain times of the year, and enhance the experiences that each season provides. These recipes are also wonderful for parties, as they're already seasonally themed!

ALL THE STONE FRUIT!

1 peach, pitted and cut into eighths
1 nectarine, pitted and quartered
1 plum, pitted and quartered
ice
1½ quarts still water

Add peaches, nectarines, and plums to the insert of a 2-quart infusion pitcher. Add desired amount of ice to pitcher, then fill with water. Allow to steep for at least 30 minutes, but preferably for 2 to 3 hours, before serving.

TIP: Other delicious stone fruit includes apricots, pluots, and cherries, so feel free to mix and match stone fruit! You can also freeze your stone fruit in the summer so that you can enjoy this infusion throughout the rest of the year.

AUGUST IN NAPA

juice and rinds of 1 lime
1½ quarts still water
1 cup strawberries, sliced
1 nectarine, sliced
10 black peppercorns, crushed
8 to 10 fresh mint leaves
1 medium rhubarb stalk, cut into to 1-inch sections
1 cup ice (optional)

Cut the lime in half, juice both halves, and reserve the rinds. Add water and lime juice to a 2-quart pitcher. In a mesh sachet, combine lime halves, strawberries, nectarine slices, crushed peppercorns, mint, and rhubarb. Place sachet in the lime water and steep for at least 30 minutes, but preferably 3 to 5 hours. Remove sachet from water, squeezing liquid back into the pitcher. Serve neat or over ice. Consider serving over Nectarine and Basil Ice Cubes (page 142) to really impress your guests!

TIP: Another preparation option for this recipe is to use an infusion pitcher and add the lime halves, strawberries, nectarines, mint, and rhubarb to the insert, then fill the pitcher with water. We still recommend adding the peppercorns to a sachet before adding to the insert, to avoid unwanted floaties in your beverage.

STRAWBERRY LIME BASIL SPRITZER

2 cups strawberries, hulled and quartered
1 lime, sliced into wheels
2 to 4 sprigs fresh basil, stems included
½ quart still water
1 quart sparkling water
ice

Add strawberries, limes, and basil to the insert of a 2-quart infusion pitcher. Add desired amount of ice to pitcher, then fill with still and sparkling water. Allow to steep for at least 30 minutes, but preferably for 2 to 3 hours, before serving in champagne flutes. Garnish each glass with a quarter of a strawberry.

TIP: Like more or less fizz? Adjust amounts of still versus sparkling water accordingly. Just make sure the still water, sparkling water, and ingredients amount to 2 quarts.

PEACH LAVENDER RELAXER

2 peaches, pitted and cut into small chunks
1 sprig fresh lavender
2 drops lavender essential oil
1½ quarts still water

Add peaches and fresh lavender to the insert of a 2-quart infusion pitcher. Add desired amount of ice to pitcher, add the essential oil, then fill with water. Allow to steep for at least 30 minutes, but preferably for 2 to 3 hours, before serving.

TIP: Because lavender is such a relaxing herb, this combo is wonderful at the end of the day as you unwind!

CRANBERRY CITRUS MOCKTAIL

1 cup fresh cranberries, halved
2 limes, 1 sliced into wheels and 1 cut into wedges
ice
2 drops orange essential oil
½ quart still water
1 quart sparkling water

Add cranberries and lime wheels to the insert of a 2-quart infusion pitcher. Add desired amount of ice to pitcher, add the essential oil and still water, then fill with sparkling water. Allow to steep for at least 30 minutes, but preferably for 2 to 3 hours, before serving. Garnish each glass with a lime wedge when serving.

TIP: To make sure your beverage is nice and fizzy, top each glass with a little more sparkling water before serving! This mocktail is a beautiful and delicious accompaniment to Thanksgiving dinner.

APPLE PIE TREAT

2 apples, cored and cut into chunks
1 medium vanilla bean, sliced lengthwise
1 cinnamon stick
1 tablespoon whole cloves
½-inch piece of fresh ginger, peeled
ice
½ quart still water
1½ quarts sparkling water

Add apples, vanilla bean, and cinnamon stick to the insert of a 2-quart infusion pitcher. Place cloves and ginger in a tea ball or sachet and add to the other ingredients. Add desired amount of ice to pitcher, add the still water, then fill with sparkling water. Allow to steep for at least 30 minutes, but preferably for 2 to 3 hours, before serving.

TIP: This fall-themed beverage is great on a cool evening, and is beautiful served with a cinnamon stick!

BLACKBERRY GRAPE INFUSION

1 cup blackberries
½ cup green seedless grapes, halved
½ cup red seedless grapes, halved
ice
1½ quarts still water

Add blackberries and grapes to the insert of a 2-quart infusion pitcher. Add desired amount of ice to pitcher, then fill with water. Allow to steep for at least 30 minutes, but preferably for 2 to 3 hours, before serving.

TIP: Fall doesn't equate with cool weather in all parts of the country! If your region enjoys a warm "Indian Summer," try freezing your blackberries and grapes before adding to your infusion for an even more refreshing beverage!

AUTUMN INFUSED GOODNESS

2 tablespoons pomegranate seeds
1 persimmon, thinly sliced
1 orange, cut into eighths
2 cinnamon sticks
1 teaspoon allspice berries
1½ quarts still water
2 drops orange essential oil

Muddle the pomegranate seeds in a pint glass to break them open, then scoop them into the base of a 2-quart infusion pitcher. Add persimmon, oranges, and cinnamon sticks to the insert. Place allspice berries in a tea ball or sachet and add to insert. Fill the pitcher with water, then add essential oil. Allow to steep for at least 30 minutes, but preferably for 2 to 3 hours, before serving. Remove allspice berries after 30 minutes, regardless of how long the rest of the mixture steeps. May be served at room temperature, chilled, or over ice.

TIP: This combination can easily make a delicious autumn mocktail—just swap still water for sparkling water!

WINTER IMMUNITY

1 green apple, cored and thinly sliced
1 crisp pear, cored and thinly sliced
1 cinnamon stick
4 cardamom seeds
1 tablespoon whole cloves
1 tablespoon lemon juice
1 drop orange essential oil
1½ quarts still water

Add apples, pears, and cinnamon stick to the insert of a 2-quart infusion pitcher. Place cardamom seeds and cloves in a tea ball or sachet and add to insert. Add lemon juice and essential oil to the pitcher, then fill with water. Allow to steep for at least 30 minutes, but preferably for 2 to 3 hours, before serving. Remove tea ball or sachet after 30 minutes, regardless of how long the rest of the mixture steeps.

TIP: The combination of orange, cinnamon, and cloves is an amazing, immune system booster!

ORANGE APPLE CINNAMON COLD BUSTER

1 large apple, cored and cut into 1-inch chunks
1 large orange, sliced into wheels
1 cinnamon stick
ice (optional)
2 drops orange essential oil
1½ quarts still water

This recipe can be served hot, room temperature, or cold. Add whichever temperature of water you desire. Add apples, oranges, and cinnamon stick to the insert of a 2-quart infusion pitcher. Add desired amount of ice to pitcher if serving cold, add the essential oil, then fill with water. Allow to steep for at least 30 minutes, but preferably for 2 to 3 hours, before serving.

TIP: If serving hot, use mugs and garnish with a cinnamon stick. If serving room temperature or cold, garnish with a slice of orange.

CITRUS BLISS

1 lemon, sliced into rounds

1 orange, sliced into rounds

1 lime, sliced into rounds

1 medium vanilla bean

2 quarts still water

1 drop grapefruit essential oil

Add lemons, oranges, limes, and vanilla bean to the insert of a 2-quart infusion pitcher. Fill pitcher with water and add essential oil. Allow to steep for at least 30 minutes, but preferably for 2 to 3 hours, before serving.

TIP: Bright citrus meets warm vanilla for this invigorating winter combo!

PEAR POMEGRANATE CLOVE MOCKTAIL

1 pear, cored and cut into 1-inch chunks
½ cup pomegranate seeds
1 tablespoon whole cloves
ice
½ quart still water
1½ quarts sparkling water

Add pears and pomegranate seeds to the insert of a 2-quart infusion pitcher. Place cloves in a tea ball or sachet and add to insert. Add desired amount of ice to pitcher, add still water, then fill with sparkling water. Allow to steep for at least 30 minutes, but preferably for 2 to 3 hours, before serving. Remove tea ball or sachet after 30 minutes, regardless how long the rest of the mixture steeps. Best served over ice in tall glasses.

TIP: Like more or less fizz? Adjust amounts of still versus sparkling water accordingly. Just make sure the still water, sparkling water, and ingredients amount to 2 quarts.

SPRING RECHARGE

1 cup blueberries

½ cup strawberries, sliced

2 oranges, sliced into wheels

2 sprigs fresh lavender (or 2 tablespoons dried lavender)

1 cup ice

2 drops orange essential oil

1½ quarts still water

Place the blueberries and strawberries in a small bowl, mash with a muddler, then add them to the base of a 2-quart infusion pitcher. Add oranges and lavender to the insert. Add ice to the pitcher, then top with essential oil, still water and sparkling water. Infuse for at least 30 minutes, but preferably for 3 to 5 hours in the refrigerator before serving. Serve chilled or over ice.

TIP: Consider serving over Summertime Ice Cubes (page 143) for even more fruit flavor!

GRAPEFRUIT MINT MOCKTAIL

2 grapefruits, cut into thick wedges
1 to 2 sprigs fresh mint
ice
½ quart still water
2 drops grapefruit essential oil
1½ quarts sparkling water

Add grapefruit and mint to the insert of a 2-quart infusion pitcher. Add desired amount of ice to pitcher, add still water and essential oil, then fill with sparkling water. Allow to steep for at least 30 minutes, but preferably for 2 to 3 hours, before serving. Serve over ice in tumblers, adding a bit more sparkling water at the time of serving. Garnish glasses with a wedge of grapefruit.

TIP: Like more or less fizz? Adjust amounts of still versus sparkling water accordingly. Just make sure the still water, sparkling water, and ingredients amount to 2 quarts.

ALL THE BERRIES!

1 cup strawberries, hulled and quartered
½ cup raspberries
½ cup blackberries
ice
1½ quarts water

Add strawberries, raspberries, and blackberries to the insert of a 2-quart infusion pitcher. Add desired amount of ice to pitcher, then fill with water. Allow to steep for at least 30 minutes, but preferably for 2 to 3 hours, before serving.

TIP: Want to enjoy berries all year? Just buy them in bulk in the springtime, then freeze for later use!

PINEAPPLE MANGO MINT COLADA

1 cup pineapple, hulled and cut into 1-inch chunks
1 cup mango, peeled, pitted, and cut into 1-inch chunks
1 to 2 sprigs fresh mint
ice
½ quart still water
1½ quarts sparkling water

Add pineapple, mangos, and mint to the insert of a 2-quart infusion pitcher. Add desired amount of ice to pitcher, add still water, then fill with sparkling water. Allow to steep for at least 30 minutes, but preferably for 2 to 3 hours, before serving. Serve over ice in tumblers and garnish each glass with a sprig of mint.

TIP: For fizzier drinks, use a regular pitcher and just cover the ingredients with still water to infuse. Then when you're ready to serve, pour mixture into glasses and top with sparkling water.

HEALING INFUSIONS

Modern medicine is derived from plants. Historically, fruits, vegetables, herbs, spices, oils, and other parts of plants have been utilized in different combinations for their healing properties. As such, we've put together a selection of recipes with distinct health goals in mind!

RECHARGE THE SENSES

5 lychees, sliced
½ cup blueberries
½ cup raspberries
1 medium vanilla bean, split lengthwise
½ cup still water
juice of 1 lime
1 drop of orange essential oil
1 quart sparkling water

Add lychees, blueberries, raspberries, and vanilla bean to the insert of a 2-quart infusion pitcher. Add still water, lime juice and essential oil to the pitcher, then fill with sparkling water. Allow to steep for at least 30 minutes, but preferably for 2 to 3 hours, before serving. May be served at room temperature, chilled, or over ice. Kick it up a notch by adding Citrus Burst Ice Cubes (page 144).

TIP: Lychee fruit helps improve blood flow, blueberries boost brain function, vanilla is comforting, and orange oil is invigorating, so this combination is a literal recharge of the senses!

MORNING REGENERATION

1 orange, sliced into wheels
1 tangerine, sliced into wheels
3 sprigs fresh mint
½ cucumber, sliced into thin wheels
1 kiwi, peeled and sliced into wheels
1½ quarts still water

Add oranges, tangerines, mint, cucumbers, and kiwi to the insert of a 2-quart infusion pitcher. Fill pitcher with water. Allow to steep for at least 30 minutes, but preferably for 2 to 3 hours, before serving.

TIP: Invigorating orange and detoxifying cucumber make this an ideal combination for getting mornings started right.

WEIGHT LOSS POWER WATER

1 Meyer lemon, sliced into wheels
1-inch piece fresh ginger, peeled and cut into 1-inch chunks
juice of ½ ruby red grapefruit
juice of 1 orange
juice of 1 Meyer lemon
1½ quarts still water
10 to 12 Lemon Mint Ice Cubes (page 140)

Add sliced lemons and ginger to the insert of a 2-quart infusion pitcher. Add grapefruit, orange, and lemon juices to the pitcher, then fill with water. Allow to steep for at least 30 minutes, but preferably for 2 to 3 hours, before serving. Serve over Lemon Mint Ice Cubes.

TIP: Grapefruit, lemon, ginger, and mint are all detoxifying metabolism boosters! So combining these ingredients in water is a healthy kickstart to any weight-loss plan.

MANGO GINGERADE

1 mango, chopped
juice of 1 lime
juice of 1 lemon
1 tablespoon fresh ginger, finely chopped
1 date, pitted and halved
pinch of salt
2 cups still water
1 quart sparkling water

Add mango, lime juice, lemon juice, ginger, date, salt, and 2 cups of still water to a blender and puree until smooth. Pour blended ingredients through a fine-mesh sieve into a 2-quart pitcher and add sparkling water. Stir well and infuse for at least 30 minutes, but preferably for 3 to 5 hours. Serve chilled or over ice. Consider serving over Spicy Pineapple Ice Cubes (page 145) to further intensify flavors!

TIP: Ginger and sparkling water can both ease an upset stomach, so this is a healthy, natural way to help tummy aches.

POST-WORKOUT REGENERATOR

½ cup blueberries
1 golden kiwi, peeled and sliced into wheels
1 cup raspberries
¼ cup young coconut meat
2 cups coconut water
1 quart still water
pinch of sea salt

Combine blueberries, kiwi, and raspberries in a bowl and mash with a muddler. Transfer muddled ingredients to the bottom of a 2-quart infusion pitcher. Add the coconut meat to the insert, then add coconut water, still water, and pinch of salt to the pitcher. Infuse in refrigerator for at least 30 minutes, but preferably for 3 to 5 hours before serving chilled or over ice. Consider serving over Summertime Ice Cubes (page 143) to boost the antioxidant power of this infusion.

TIP: Hydration is always important, especially after working out! Sweating allows for the release of toxins, along with the excretion of water and electrolytes. This combination of antioxidants in the fruit and coconut allows for maximum replenishment.

SUPER BERRY ANTIOXIDANT BOOST

½ cup blueberries
½ cup blackberries
½ cup raspberries
½ cup cherries, halved and pitted
¼ small red beet, peeled and chopped
1 quart plus 2 cups still water

Combine blueberries, blackberries, raspberries, cherries, beet, and 2 cups of the water to a blender and blend until smooth, approximately 1 minute. Pour blended ingredients through a fine-mesh sieve into a 2-quart pitcher and add the remaining water. Refrigerate infusion for at least 30 minutes before serving chilled or over ice.

TIP: To modify this recipe for use with an infusion pitcher, just add the fruit and beets to the insert, then fill with pitcher with water. The blended version allows for greater nutrition mixed into the water, but using an infusion pitcher provides a quick and healthy alternative!

REFRESH & RENEW QUENCHER

1 lemon, sliced into wheels

1½ quarts still water

2 drops lemon essential oil

1 drop peppermint essential oil

12 Lemon Mint Ice Cubes (page 140)

Add lemons to the insert of a 2-quart infusion pitcher. Fill pitcher with water and add essential oils. Allow to steep for at least 30 minutes, but preferably for 2 to 3 hours, before serving. Serve over Lemon Mint Ice Cubes.

TIP: The combination of lemon and peppermint is extremely refreshing. This combination is perfect for a super-hot day or an afternoon pick-me-up.

CRANBERRY DETOX SPARKLER

¾ cup fresh or frozen cranberries
1 apple, cored and chopped
juice of 1 lemon
zest of ½ orange
1 cup still water
2 tablespoons pomegranate seeds
2 quarts sparkling water
orange peel (for garnish)

Combine cranberries, apple, orange zest, lemon juice, and still water in a blender and blend until smooth, approximately 1 minute. Pour blended mixture through a fine-mesh sieve into a 2-quart pitcher. Add pomegranate seeds and sparkling water, then stir and serve with orange peel garnish. To intensify flavors, refrigerate infusion for 2 hours before serving.

TIP: Want to modify this recipe to use your infusion pitcher? Just add ingredients to the insert and fill the pitcher with still and/or sparkling water.

LEAN GREEN MACHINE

½ cup spinach leaves
juice of 1 lemon
1 cup still water
1 kiwi, peeled and sliced into wheels
3 to 4 sprigs fresh parsley
8 to 10 fresh mint leaves
1 lime, sliced into wheels
1½ quarts sparkling water

Combine spinach, lemon juice, and 1 cup of the still water in the blender and blend until smooth, approximately 1 minute. Pour mixture through a fine-mesh sieve into the bottom of a 2-quart infusion pitcher. Add kiwi, parsley, mint and lime wheels to the insert. Fill the pitcher with sparkling water. Refrigerate infusion for 2 hours to intensify flavors before serving.

TIP: Adding the blended spinach to your infusion will add a serving of veggies to your beverage, with very few additional calories.

VITAL REJUVENATION

2 cups watermelon, cubed
½ cucumber, sliced into rounds
1 lemon, sliced into wheels
5 sprigs fresh cilantro
2 sprigs fresh mint
1½ quarts still water
pinch of salt
1 drop peppermint essential oil

Add watermelon, cucumbers, lemons, cilantro, and mint to the insert of a 2-quart infusion pitcher. Fill the pitcher with water and add the essential oil and pinch of salt. Allow to steep for at least 30 minutes, but preferably for 2 to 3 hours, before serving. Consider serving over Lemon Mint Ice Cubes (page 140) for even more hydrating power!

TIP: Cucumber, lemon, and peppermint are all detoxifying, whereas the watermelon and salt provide a balance of electrolytes to the mix. The combination is rejuvenating.

SUBLIME PINEAPPLE FLUSH

2 cups fresh or frozen pineapple, cut into chunks, divided
juice of 1 lime
juice of ½ lemon
2 quarts plus 1 cup still water, divided
3-inch piece fresh ginger, peeled and cut into 1-inch chunks
2 drops lime essential oil
pinch of salt

Add 1 cup of the pineapple, lime juice, lemon juice, and 1 cup of the water to a blender and blend until smooth, approximately 1 minute. Pour blended mixture through a fine-mesh sieve into the base of a 2-quart infusion pitcher. Add remaining pineapple and ginger to the insert. Fill pitcher with water, add essential oil and pinch of salt. Refrigerate infusion for 2 hours before serving, and consider serving over Spicy Pineapple Ice Cubes (page 145) for an additional metabolic boost!

TIP: Ginger helps boost metabolism as well as aid digestion, and the fiber in pineapple helps with elimination, which is why this combination is great for flushing our your system!

BODY RESTORE

1 carrot, chopped
1 celery stalk, chopped
juice of 1 lemon
1 green apple, cored and chopped
3-inch piece fresh ginger, peeled and cut into 1-inch chunks
2 quarts plus 1 cup still water

Add carrot, celery, lemon juice, and 1 cup of the water to a blender and blend until smooth, approximately 1 minute. Pour blended mixture through a fine-mesh sieve into the base of a 2-quart infusion pitcher. Add the apple and ginger to the insert, then fill the pitcher with water. Refrigerate infusion for 2 hours before serving.

TIP: Blending veggies before adding to the mixture ensures their maximum health benefit seeps right into the infusion. The combination of fruit, veggies, and ginger provides an excellent balance of vitamin, minerals, and metabolism boost!

STRESS-REDUCING TONIC

2 cups fresh or frozen pineapple, cut into chunks
juice of 1 lemon
1½ quarts plus 1 cup still water, divided
1 ruby red grapefruit, sliced into rounds
2 sprigs fresh rosemary
2 drops grapefruit essential oil

Add pineapple, lemon juice and 1 cup of the water to a blender and blend until smooth, approximately 1 minute. Pour mixture through a fine-mesh sieve into the bottom of a 2-quart infusion pitcher. Add grapefruit and rosemary to the insert, then fill pitcher with remaining water and essential oil. Infuse in the refrigerator for at least 30 minutes, but preferably 2 to 3 hours before serving.

Grapefruit helps in lowering blood pressure and boosting metabolism, both of which can help reduce the toxic effects that stress can have on the body!

RELAXING HERB SIPPER

2 sprigs fresh rosemary
2 sprigs fresh lavender
1 cup seedless green grapes
1 orange, sliced into wheels
2 quarts still water
juice of 1 lemon
2 drops lemon essential oil
1 drop lavender essential oil
ice, to serve

Add rosemary, lavender, grapes, and oranges to the insert of a 2-quart infusion pitcher. Fill the pitcher with water and add the lemon juice and essential oils. Allow to steep for at least 30 minutes, but preferably for 2 to 3 hours, before serving.

TIP: This calming blend is perfect at the end of a long day as a way to unwind before bedtime. Combine with a hot bath and soothing music and you'll drift easily into dreamland!

SWEET SERENITY

1½ tablespoons dried lavender

4 fresh sage leaves

2 teaspoons dried hibiscus flowers

2 teaspoons dried chamomile flowers

1 teaspoon dried lemon peel

1½ quarts still water

Combine lavender, sage, hibiscus, chamomile, and lemon peel in a tea ball or sachet, then add to the insert of a 2-quart infusion pitcher. Fill the pitcher with water and infuse for 3 to 5 hours before serving. Consider serving over Crimson Flower Ice Cubes (page 141) for a color burst!

TIP: Because all of the ingredients in this recipe are dried, it's best to use a tea ball or sachet in addition to the insert in an infusion pitcher to avoid having any little pieces floating in your beverage! This combination is very calming and relaxing, resembling an herbal tea.

VITAMIN C REPLENISHMENT

1 blood orange, sliced into wheels
1 medium vanilla bean, sliced lengthwise
1 teaspoon cardamom seeds
1½ quarts still water
1 teaspoon lemon juice
juice of 1 blood orange
1 drop orange essential oil

Add oranges and vanilla bean to the insert of a 2-quart infusion pitcher. Place the cardamom seeds in a tea ball or sachet and add to the insert. Fill the pitcher with water and add the lemon juice, blood orange juice, and essential oil. Allow to steep for at least 30 minutes, but preferably for 2 to 3 hours, before serving.

TIP: Oranges and lemons are both exceptionally high in vitamin C, a nutrient that plays an important role in the formation and healing of tissues in the body, as well as in the function of the immune system. This combination is a great immune boost to drink if you feel a bit run down or like a cold is coming on.

IMMUNITY & CLARITY BOOSTER

1 mango, peeled, pitted, and chopped
juice of 1 lime
juice of 1 orange
1½ quarts plus 1 cup still water, divided
8 sprigs fresh cilantro
1 kiwi, peeled and sliced into wheels

Combine mango, lime juice, orange juice, and 1 cup of water in a blender and blend until smooth, approximately 1 minute. Pour blended mixture through a fine-mesh sieve into the bottom of a 2-quart infusion pitcher. Add cilantro and kiwi to the insert, then fill pitcher with remaining water. Refrigerate for 2 to 3 hours before serving over ice.

TIP: Like citrus fruit, cilantro is high in vitamin C, making it an excellent herb for boosting immune system function!

SUPREME CIRCULATION TONIC

1 plum, pitted and chopped
juice of 1 orange
½ teaspoon ground cinnamon
1½ quarts plus 1 cup still water, divided
½ cup blackberries
½ cup cherries, pitted and halved
1 cinnamon stick

Combine plums, orange juice, ground cinnamon, and 1 cup of water into a blender and blend until smooth, approximately 1 minute. Pour blended mixture through a fine-mesh sieve into the bottom of a 2-quart infusion pitcher. Add blackberries, cherries, and cinnamon stick to the insert, then fill pitcher with remaining water. Refrigerate infusion for 3 to 5 hours before serving over ice.

TIP: Cherries and cinnamon both boast improved circulation in their lists of health benefits, so this is an excellent combination for improvement lymphatic and blood circulation in the body.

YOUTHFUL TONIC

2 cups watermelon, cubed
10 fresh basil leaves
½ cup fresh young coconut meat
1½ quarts still water
1 tablespoon lemon juice
2 drops lemon essential oil
pinch of sea salt

Add watermelon, basil, and coconut to the insert of a 2-quart infusion pitcher. Fill the pitcher with water and add the lemon juice, essential oil, and pinch of salt. Allow to steep for at least 30 minutes, but preferably for 2 to 3 hours, before serving.

TIP: Lemon is a great detoxifier, and its use over time improves the look and feel of skin dramatically.

DETOX & SKIN RENEWAL

½ cup blueberries
1 lemon, sliced into wheels
½ cucumber, sliced into rounds
1½ quarts still water
2 drops lemon essential oil

In a small bowl, mash blueberries. Add muddled blueberries to the base of a 2-quart infusion pitcher. Add lemons and cucumbers to the insert, then fill pitcher with water and essential oil. Refrigerate infusion for 3 to 5 hours before serving.

TIP: Give your skin a drink of water with this detoxifying infusion. This is a great combination to drink before or after a workout.

ICE CUBE RECIPES

Infused ice cubes are great for adding to plain still or sparkling water, or to infused water recipes! They're quick and easy to make, and allow for storing for later use. Just as with infusion recipes, ingredients can be mixed and matched. We've found these combinations to stand out on their own as well as complement many of the other recipes in the book. Infused ice cubes are especially impressive at parties!

LEMON MINT ICE CUBES

¼ cup lemon juice
1 cup fresh mint leaves
2½ cups still water

Combine lemon juice, mint leaves, and water in a blender and blend until smooth, approximately 1 minute. Pour mixture into ice cube trays and freeze.

TIP: Lemon and mint ice cubes are meant to dress up many of our infusion recipes in the book. These ice cubes are very cool and refreshing, and pair best with citrus infusions.

CRIMSON FLOWER ICE CUBES

2 tablespoons dried hibiscus tea flowers
3 cups hot still water
3 tablespoons pomegranate seeds

Steep dried hibiscus flowers in 3 cups hot water for 4 to 5 minutes, until the water changes color. Pour mixture into a glass pitcher and refrigerate for at least 30 minutes to cool. Once the mixture is cooled, pour into standard ice cube trays. Add a few pomegranate seeds to each cube well and freeze. There should be enough mixture to fill two ice cube trays.

TIP: These beautiful ice cubes will add a pop of bright crimson color to any water infusion. They are perfect for parties and holiday events.

NECTARINE & BASIL ICE CUBES

2 nectarines, pitted
juice of 1 lemon
2 cups still water
4 fresh basil leaves, julienned

Add nectarines, lemon juice, and water to a blender and blend until smooth, approximately 1 minute. Pour mixture through a fine-mesh sieve into a pitcher, and add the julienned basil strips. Mix well, then pour into standard ice cube trays, making sure that some basil gets into each cube well. Freeze and enjoy.

TIP: These ice cubes are perfect to enjoy during the summer, on a hot day with a nice picnic. Adding these ice cubes to any seasonal summer infusion will provide more flavor and complexity.

SUMMERTIME ICE CUBES

½ cup blueberries
1 kiwi, peeled, sliced into wheels and then quartered
24 seedless green grapes, halved
2 cups still water

Place a blueberry, 2 kiwi pieces, and a grape half into each cube well of a standard ice cube tray. Pour water to fill each cube well. Freeze and enjoy.

TIP: These ice cubes add just the right amount of color and fun to many of our water infusions. Receive an extra antioxidant boost with these cubes and enjoy as they melt in your water.

CITRUS BURST ICE CUBES

juice of 1 lemon
juice of 1 orange
2 cups still water
12 pieces orange peel

Blend lemon juice, orange juice, and water in a blender until smooth, approximately 30 seconds. Place a piece of orange peel into each ice cube well of a standard ice cube tray. Then fill each cube well with blended mixture and freeze.

TIP: The perfect way to add more citrus power to your water is with these flavorful ice cubes. They pair with citrus water infusions along with infusions for the fall and winter seasons.

SPICY PINEAPPLE ICE CUBES

2 cups fresh pineapple, diced
juice of 1 lime
2 cups still water
1 jalapeño, seeded and sliced into thin wheels

Add pineapple, lime juice, and water to a blender and blend until smooth, approximately 1 minute. Place 1 to 2 jalapeño wheels into each cube well of a standard ice cube tray. Pour blended mixture into tray and freeze.

TIP: Add a kick to your water with these tangy, spicy pineapple ice cubes. They are perfectly paired with Latin-inspired dishes.

CONVERSION CHARTS

COMMON CONVERSIONS

1 gallon = 4 quarts = 8 pints = 16 cups = 128 fluid ounces = 3.8 liters
1 quart = 2 pints = 4 cups = 32 ounces = .95 liter
1 pint = 2 cups = 16 ounces = 480 ml
1 cup = 8 ounces = 240 ml
¼ cup = 4 tablespoons = 12 teaspoons = 2 ounces = 60 ml
1 tablespoon = 3 teaspoons = ½ fluid ounce = 15 ml

TEMPERATURE CONVERSIONS

FAHRENHEIT (°F)	CELSIUS (°C)
200°F	95°C
225°F	110°C
250°F	120°C
275°F	135°C
300°F	150°C
325°F	165°C
350°F	175°C
375°F	190°C
400°F	200°C
425°F	220°C
450°F	230°C
475°F	245°C

VOLUME CONVERSIONS

U.S.	U.S. EQUIVALENT	METRIC
1 tablespoon (3 teaspoons)	½ fluid ounce	15 milliliters
¼ cup	2 fluid ounces	60 milliliters
⅓ cup	3 fluid ounces	90 milliliters
½ cup	4 fluid ounces	120 milliliters
⅔ cup	5 fluid ounces	150 milliliters
¾ cup	6 fluid ounces	180 milliliters
1 cup	8 fluid ounces	240 milliliters
2 cups	16 fluid ounces	480 milliliters

WEIGHT CONVERSIONS

U.S.	METRIC
½ ounce	15 grams
1 ounce	30 grams
2 ounces	60 grams
¼ pound	115 grams
⅓ pound	150 grams
½ pound	225 grams
¾ pound	350 grams
1 pound	450 grams

RECIPE INDEX

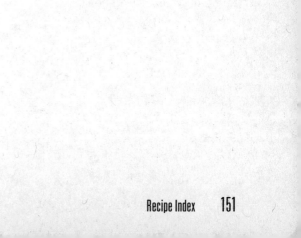

ACKNOWLEDGMENTS

To our patients, clients, team members, publisher, friends, and most importantly our husbands...thank you.

ABOUT THE AUTHORS

This healthy nutrition book is the fourth collaboration of Drs. Mariza Snyder and Lauren Clum. Their other works include *The Antioxidant Counter: A Pocket Guide to the Revolutionary ORAC Scale for Choosing Healthy Foods*, *The DASH Diet Cookbook: Quick and Delicious Recipes for Losing Weight, Preventing Diabetes and Lowering Blood Pressure*, and *The Low-GI Slow Cooker: Delicious and Easy Dishes Made Healthy with the Glycemic Index*.

Dr. Mariza Snyder is a passionate and dedicated wellness practitioner and speaker committed to inspiring people to live a healthy and abundant life through plant-based nutrition and simple lifestyle changes.

Dr. Lauren Clum is a chiropractor with The Specific Chiropractic Center, practicing in Oakland, California. Since opening her practice in 2007 she has been dedicated to standing out as a trustworthy resource to her community, advocating for truth and fairness in health and healing.